CREATE THE LIFE YOU WANT:
FEEL FABULOUS INSIDE OUT

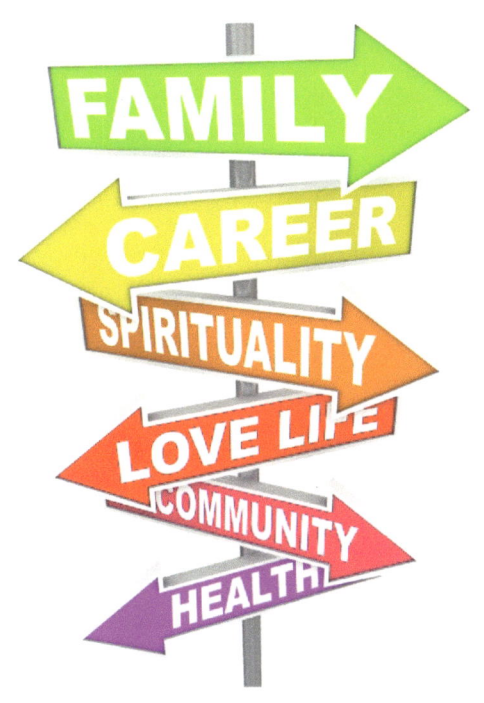

ANGELA BOYD

CREATE THE LIFE YOU WANT

DEDICATION

This book is dedicated to my children, Kenya, Andrew and Kenneth who are the driving force in everything I do. They are the reason why I have been on this physical and mental journey to health and wellness. I want them to live and create their best life according to their true purpose and calling.

CREATE THE LIFE YOU WANT

*You are the designer of
your destiny. You are
the author of your story.*

~Lisa Nichols

TABLE OF CONTENTS

INTRODUCTION 3
  WHY IS IT IMPORTANT TO BE HEALTHY 3
CHAPTER 1 5
  SELF CARE...5
    RELATIONSHIPS 5
    CAREER..6
    EXERCISE 7
    SELF CARE STRATEGIES...8
CHAPTER 2..13
  HEALTHY FOOD CHOICES 13
    GRAINS 17
    BEANS 19
    OILS...19
    PROTEINS..22
    PROTECT YOUR BONES...24
CHAPTER 3..27
  HAVE MORE ENERGY 27
CHAPTER 4..29
  READ YOUR LABELS 29
CHAPTER 5..31
  NO MORE SUGAR BLUES...31
    EAT LESS SUGAR, FEEL ALIVE...32
    WHAT'S WRONG WITH SUGAR 33
    THE MANY NAMES OF SUGAR...34
    ARTIFICIAL SWEETENERS..34
    WAYS TO KEEP YOUR BLOOD SUGAR STEADY 35
CHAPTER 6..37
  NUTRITIOUS SNACKS 37
    LIST OF HEALTHY SNACKS..37
    BAD MOOD FOODS..38
CHAPTER 7..39
  SUPER FOODS FOR A SUPER BODY 39
CHAPTER 8..43
  DETOX, CLEANSING AND FASTING................................43

5 SIMPLE WAYS TO REDUCE YOUR TOXIC EXPOSURE 44

CHAPTER 9...47

PROCESS OF ELIMINATION: DIGESTIVE HEALTH........47

NATURAL WAYS TO FACILITATE ELIMINATION 47

IMMUNE SUPPORT 49

TRACK YOUR PROGRESS...51

SHOPPING LIST GUIDE...52

REFERENCES 53

ABOUT THE AUTHOR...56

ACKNOWLEDGEMENT

I would like to acknowledge my children, mother, grandmother and other family and friends who supported my efforts in writing this book. Their insight, opinions and suggestions were most helpful when I sought second opinions and comments. Lastly but not least, I'd like to thank my editor, Geogina Chong-You, who at the final stages used her meticulous eye to bring this project to completion.

Stay Positive

Take a deep breath,
keep moving forward and
don't look back.
Everything is working out
for your highest good.
Embrace and trust the process.

~ Simple Reminders

INTRODUCTION
WHY IS IT IMPORTANT TO BE HEALTHY

My personal motivation for being healthy came from my yearly visits to the doctor. During these visits my doctor issued several major concerns related to blood pressure, thyroid, weight, and energy. The doctor warned me that I would need to take prescription medication if the next check-up did not show improvement. Since I did not like to take pills, I decided to make it my mission to turn things around. My approach was to keep a food journal and write down the foods that I ate and how they made me feel. I did not think that I was eating extremely unhealthy, but actually I was. I knew I **had** to make improvements or my health was going to get worse not better. When I returned to the doctor a year later she asked me what I was doing differently, I told her that I was making much better food and lifestyle choices and that I was studying to become a health coach. After my success I decided that I wanted to help others through the same challenges I had experienced so that they too could make better decisions for their health and overall wellbeing.

As I think about my motivation and the goals I set for myself during that journey it made me think back to when I was younger.

As a child and young adult, the last thing that I was concerned about was losing weight or even my health because I always felt that I was in good health. In school, I was active and played sports with no problems. I had no major health issues and was healthy. A cold one or two times a year and a few headaches were the only issues that came up. As I have gotten older, I have learned not to take my health for granted.

Now I have to be conscious of what I eat, think and do, because it all affects how I feel mentally, physically and spiritually. Basically, they affect every aspect of my overall health.

Now, when I set goals or make decisions to do things, I think about the outcome first and the overall impact that it will have on me not just for today. Daily behavior is cumulative and has long-term consequences.

I have decided to, "Create The Life I Want to Live". It is a choice that I have made and you can too. With knowledge and awareness, we can make informed decisions and the best choices for ourselves, in the areas of health and wellness. No matter how old or young it's never too late to make a change for self-improvement.

My focus now is living a healthy balanced life. It is a choice we can all make when informed with research-based knowledge. I want to share with you what I have learned, so that you can feel your best too.

So, ask yourself, "What is my motivation for living a healthy and balanced life?" Is it to feel good inside and outside of my body?

- To live a longer life?
- To be more active?
- To eliminate a chronic disease?
- To have more energy?
- To eat better quality foods?
- To feel good all the time?

The list can go on and on, and if you think about it, we all have reasons for the things that we do. You choose your motivation and you can work toward achieving your goals. However, your motivation needs to be yours, not what someone else wants you to achieve. My motivation for being healthy is to feel good inside and out.

CHAPTER 1
SELF CARE

What I have learned is that eating healthy starts with looking at all areas of life. According to Joshua Rosenthal, the founder of the Institute for Integrative Nutrition, "First, it's important to look beyond what you are actually eating." [1]

The primary foods are the first and foremost areas that we need to focus on as we begin the journey into a healthier lifestyle. Primary foods, which are not even foods, are relationships, exercise, career and spiritual practice.

I call this focus a journey because of all of the twist and turns one must experience as we try new life style practices and foods. Basic areas to consider:

- Do you have healthy relationships with others such as family, friends, and co-workers?
- Do you exercise, walk, yoga, run, cycle or swim?
- Are you in a career that you enjoy?
- Does your life have direction and meaning?
- Do you meditate or have a spiritual practice?

Once you have thought about these questions, let's look in-depth at those areas of your life that require attention for a healthier lifestyle. They are areas that will impact your daily schedule and routines.

RELATIONSHIPS

In order to move on with your life or even to change certain aspects of your life, all your relationships need to be in alignment, so to speak. If there are one or two friendships that are unsettled or that have ended without closure, they need to be sorted out so you can move on with your life. Each relationship that we have may be different, but they are all important in our life. Build them with care.

A relationship that is unsettled keeps your mind occupied with thoughts of what you might have said or what you would say now in hindsight. It will engage your mind with questions of how you could have handled it better or what you should not have said to your friend. It is suggested that you need to either end the relationship completely or patch the friendship.

It's the same with family members with whom you may not have a good relationship due to many things including betrayals, trust, or personality conflicts. Ending or mending a relationship allows you to move on to another place in your life.

Relationships are key to knowing, sustaining and being involved in your community. It is through community with others that we fulfill our purpose, maintain balance and find meaning in caring about those around us. Many times it is because we find strength in serving others that we can move past obstacles and achieve our goals.

CAREER

Your career occupies a large portion of your daily life. It is an important aspect of your wellbeing. Having a job that is so stressful you can't sleep at night has a negative impact your health. The body regenerates during sleep, so you need proper rest of at least seven to eight hours of sleep every night if you want to function properly the following day.

You need to take a good look at your career and determine if it's going where you want it to go; or it may be time to look for another career or a different company. There are some people who keep a job believing there isn't another one that will give them the security they need, especially in today's economy. However, if you take the time and with proper search techniques, you might find another career that will work hand-in-hand with your health and family.

It takes courage to make the decision to move on to another job. It is a big risk, but sometimes it's necessary for your health and lifestyle. The body can only take so much stress before the stress shows up in different ways or some disease takes over due to your body's weak immune system.

EXERCISE

Exercise brings about balance in your health. Without exercise, your body is at high risk for many preventable illnesses and it can accelerate the aging process. Believe it or not, an inactive body is a negative body, mind and soul. Exercise is necessary for your body to stay in shape, keep the muscles toned to energize the mind and deliver oxygen and nutrients throughout the body.

Your mind will sharpen when you exercise at least three times a week. Exercise releases chemicals in the form of hormones and enzymes in the body to trigger emotions that rule your life. It doesn't have to be hours of workouts at the gym; it can be an extra trip up the stairs, or a long walk around the block, or even riding your bike several miles a day and my favorite, yoga stretches in the morning.

These exercises help keep the body and mind toned and in balance. They strip away stress and tension and allow you to relax without worry.

It is important to focus on health and wellness because your overall quality of life depends on it to function at its best.

SELF CARE STRATEGIES

Increasing self-care is one of the best ways to improve how you feel. Your overall outlook on life and even your energy level will peak as you engage in daily self-care activities. When you do things to take care of yourself, which include the things that you are passionate about, it fuels your soul.

When you allow yourself to take a break and relax, you feel refreshed and have renewed energy as well. Nourishing your soul by making healthy choices will invigorate and motivate you to a new level of overall effectiveness.

Here are a few tips to remain calm and reduce stress:

- Eat the best and most nutritious foods
  Choose more fruits and vegetables, drink more water, and choose whole foods.

- Exercise
  Exercise regularly, especially cardiovascular exercises to release endorphins, which are feel-good hormones.

- Relax
  Manage stress holistically using relaxation techniques that are easy to integrate into a daily routine such as yoga, meditation and breathing exercises. Find one that resonates with you. Yoga can be great to help release hormones that are conducive to relaxation. It is a way to encourage conscious and deep breathing, and using hip-opening poses that release stored stress and emotions.

• Write
Journaling (keeping a diary) allows you to write down what's on your mind. Many times we overthink situations in our lives and we talk ourselves into and out of things. When you multitask and have a lot of responsibilities, journaling is a quick method of expressing what you're thinking and how you're feeling. I have not always been really good about journaling. I tend to pick up journaling when I have a lot going on and want to capture my thoughts and feelings. When I'm not really in the mood to talk to anyone, but want to reflect on how I'm feeling, journaling gives me a chance to put what's on my mind on paper. It is very therapeutic as well. Writing about anger, sadness and other painful emotions help to release the feelings. It can make you feel calmer and better able to concentrate.

Scientific evidence supports journaling as providing many unexpected benefits. The act of writing accesses your left-brain, which is analytical and rational. While your left-brain is occupied, your right brain is free to create and feel.

Writing removes mental blocks and allows you to use all of your brainpower to better understand yourself, others and the world around you. Begin journaling and begin experiencing the benefits. Do you ever seem to feel scattered jumbled up inside, unsure of what you want or feel, or need to clarify your thoughts and feelings? Take a few minutes to write down your thoughts and emotions to discover what is going on inside. By writing routinely you will get to know what makes you feel happy and confident. You will also become clearer about situations and people who are toxic in your life. This is important information for your emotional well-being.

- Stop multi-tasking
  Try to focus on one thing at a time. Think about prioritizing and concentrating when there are multiple tasks in your schedule. It helps you become more efficient, focused, and productive.

- Go Slow
  Slow down and smell the roses! Often when you stop running in circles, you find the way out. It is important to schedule quiet time every day – even if it's just five or ten minutes. Close the door, dim the lights, turn off the computer, and silence the phone. Take these few precious minutes to do what feels good to you and recharge your battery. Notice how you feel when you are about to get into a "burn out" state, and give yourself a break before you begin to get to that state.

- Daily Positive Affirmation\Scripture
  Affirmations are phrases that are positive and can be used for self-improvement. Select your favorite for daily meditation.

- Be Grateful
  Be grateful for everything from the moment you wake up, such as your spiritual practice, family, friends, career, food, house, car...the list can go on. The more gratitude you practice the more happiness you bring into your life.

  Remember, throughout the day to say, "Thank You" for where you are -- no matter what is going on in your life.

The last tip...

• Get enough sleep
Getting enough sleep is very important. It reduces stress on the body, physically, and mentally.

Helpful tips to get a restful night sleep:

•Exercise in the morning, afternoon or evening. It is important for relaxation.

• Eliminate late night eating stop eating two to three hours before you go to sleep at night. Your body has to break down the food and the process can keep you awake and alert.

• Listen to soft music; music without words, instrumentals can be relaxing.

• Stay calm and start winding down an hour or two before bedtime.

• Practice a bedtime ritual. It can help you wind down and signal your body that it's time to relax and get ready for sleep - turn off the TV, computer or any screens at least an hour before going to bed; have a warm cup of chamomile tea, or read a book.

• Keep a notepad and pencil beside your bed for those who tend to remember things or come up with ideas around bedtime. You can write them down before going to sleep and not have to worry about whether you will remember when you wake up.

• Eliminate sugar, caffeine and alcohol prior to bedtime - they can all affect your sleep.

I
have decided to be happy ,
because it is
good for my
health.

∼unknown

CHAPTER 2
HEALTHY FOOD CHOICES

Eating fruits, vegetables, grains, beans, oils, protein and calcium supplies the body with important nutrients you need to function properly.

I remember hearing as a small child, "You must eat your vegetables." Growing up on a farm, vegetables were eaten at almost every meal. There was no question about whether you were going to eat your vegetables -- it was expected by all. I loved vegetables as a child and continue to today.

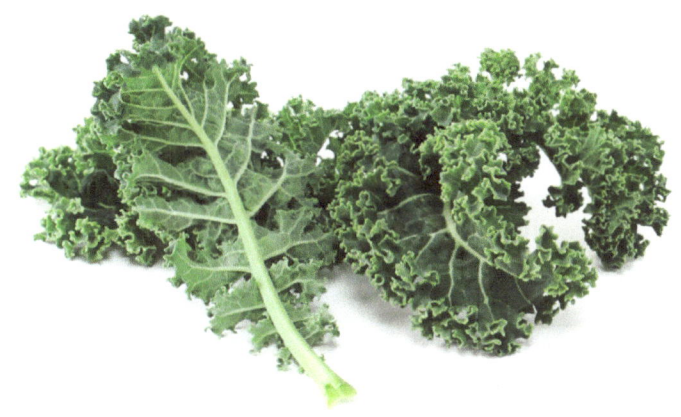

As society has changed, so has our selection of foods and their availability and easy access. Conveniences are taking priority over what is important. There are so many benefits to be gained from eating vegetables and fruits. They are great for healing, and giving you energy. They make you feel **alive!** All plants have vitamins, fiber, water, minerals, phytochemicals, and antioxidants.

According to Dr. Mark Furham in *Eat to Live* [2]; the recommendation is that our diet should consist of mostly vegetables, which he refers to as GBOMBS – greens, beans onions, mushrooms, berries and seeds. He states that the disease-fighting foods are green leafy vegetables, green peppers, and mushrooms. Whether you are having fresh fruit for a light early morning breakfast, a midday snack or evening treat, enjoy nature's sweetness and whenever possible, buy organic.

Foods contain nutrients that heal our bodies and help us maintain optimal health. However, processed foods are loaded with chemicals but deficient in nutrients. Processed foods tend to make the body crave that which has been eaten and contributes to overeating and a growing concern today called obesity.

Obesity is not only a condition of gaining unwanted weight, but it also makes you sluggish, which means your brain is not functioning at its optimal level. You may have trouble making decisions, thinking clearly, or you might even suffer from brain fog, which is caused by too much table sugar and not enough glucose. Glucose is important to proper brain functions and if you eat too much processed food, little of the energy or glucose gets to the brain. That's why it's important to eat as many fresh fruits and vegetables as you can. They have all the nutrients the body needs.

A sample list of healthy foods and their benefits:

Apples	Protects your heart	Prevents constipation	Blocks diarrhea	Improves lung capacity	Cushions joints
Apricots	Combats cancer	Controls blood pressure	Saves your eyesight	Shields against Alzheimer's	Slows aging process
Artichokes	Aids digestion	Lowers cholesterol	Protects your heart	Stabilizes blood sugar	Guards against liver disease
Avocados	Battles diabetes	Lowers cholesterol	Helps stops strokes	Controls blood pressure	Soothes skin

Bananas	Protects your heart	Quiets a cough	Strengthens bones	Controls blood pressure	Blocks diarrhea
Beans	Prevents constipation	Helps hemorrhoids	Lowers cholesterol	Combats cancer	Stabilizes blood sugar
Beets	Controls blood pressure	Combats cancer	Strengthens bones	Protects your heart	Aids weight loss
Blueberries	Combats cancer	Protects your heart	Stabilizes blood sugar	Boosts memory	Prevents constipation
Broccoli	Strengthens bones	Saves eyesight	Combats cancer	Protects your heart	Controls blood pressure
Cabbage	Combats cancer	Prevents constipation	Promotes weight loss	Protects your heart	Helps hemorrhoids
Cantaloupe	Saves eyesight	Controls blood pressure	Lowers cholesterol	Combats cancer	Supports immune system
Carrots	Saves eyesight	Protects your heart	Prevents constipation	Combats cancer	Promotes weight loss
Cauliflower	Protects against prostate cancer	Combats breast cancer	Strengthens bones	Banishes bruises	Guards against heart disease
Cherries	Protects your heart	Combats cancer	Ends insomnia	Slows aging process	Shields against Alzheimer's
Chestnuts	Promotes weight loss	Protects your heart	Lowers cholesterol	Combats cancer	Controls blood pressure
Chili peppers	Aids digestion	Soothes sore throat	Clears sinuses	Combats cancer	Boosts immune system
Figs	Promotes weight loss	Helps stops strokes	Lowers cholesterol	Combats cancer	Controls blood pressure
Fish	Protects your heart	Boosts memory	Protects your heart	Combats cancer	Supports immune system
Flax	Aids digestion	Battles diabetes	Protects your heart	Improves mental health	Boosts immune system
Garlic	Lowers cholesterol	Controls blood pressure	Combats cancer	Kills bacteria	Fights fungus
Grapefruit	Protects against heart attacks	Promotes weight loss	Helps stops strokes	Combats prostate cancer	Lowers cholesterol
Grapes	Saves eyesight	Conquers kidney stones	Combats cancer	Enhances blood flow	Protects your heart
Green tea	Combats cancer	Protects your heart	Helps stops strokes	Promotes weight loss	Kills bacteria
Honey	Heals wounds	Aids digestion	Guards against ulcers	Increases energy	Fights allergies

CREATE THE LIFE YOU WANT

Lemons	Combats cancer	Protects your heart	Controls blood pressure	Soothes skin	detox
Limes	Combats cancer	Protects your heart	Controls blood pressure	Soothes skin	Stops scurvy
Mangoes	Combats cancer	Boosts memory	Regulates thyroid	Aids digestion	Shields against Alzheimer's
Mushrooms	Controls blood pressure	Lowers cholesterol	Kills bacteria	Combats cancer	Strengthens bones
Oats	Lowers cholesterol	Combats cancer	Battles diabetes	Prevents constipation	Soothes skin
Olive oil	Protects your heart	Promotes weight loss	Combats cancer	Battles diabetes	Soothes skin
Onions	Reduce risk of heart attack	Combats cancer	Kills bacteria	Lowers cholesterol	Fights fungus
Oranges	Supports immune systems	Combats cancer	Protects your heart	Good source of fiber	Loaded with Vitamin C
Peaches	Prevents constipation	Combats cancer	Helps stops strokes	Aids digestion	Helps hemorrhoids
Peanuts	Protects against heart disease	Promotes weight loss	Combats prostate cancer	Lowers cholesterol	Aggravates diverticulitis
Pineapple	Strengthens bones	Relieves colds	Aids digestion	Dissolves warts	Blocks diarrhea
Prunes	Slows aging process	Prevents constipation	Boosts memory	Lowers cholesterol	Protects against heart disease
Rice	Protects your heart	Battles diabetes	Conquers kidney stones	Combats cancer	Helps stops strokes
Strawberries	Combats cancer	Protects your heart	Boosts memory	Calms stress	Loaded with anti-oxidants
Sweet potatoes	Saves your eyesight	Lifts mood	Combats cancer	Strengthens bones	Contains collagen
Tomatoes	Protects prostate	Combats cancer	Lowers cholesterol	Protects your heart	Loaded with vitamin C
Walnuts	Lowers cholesterol	Combats cancer	Boosts memory	Lifts mood	Protects against heart disease
Water	Promotes weight loss	Combats cancer	Conquers kidney stones	Soothes skin	Helps the organs work properly

Watermelon	Protects prostate	Promotes weight loss	Lowers cholesterol	Helps stops strokes	Controls blood pressure
Wheat germ	Combats colon cancer	Prevents constipation	Lowers cholesterol	Helps stops strokes	Improves digestion
Wheat bran	Combats colon cancer	Prevents constipation	Lowers cholesterol	Helps stops strokes	Improves digestion
Yogurt	Guards against ulcers	Strengthens bones	Lowers cholesterol	Supports immune systems	Aids in digestion

GRAINS

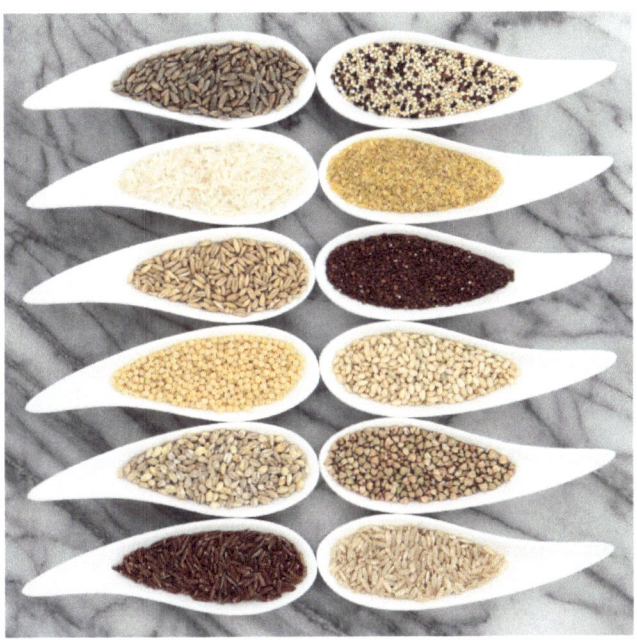

This is a list of a variety of grains and the health benefits of the most common grains.

Amaranth - is the only grain that contains vitamin C.
Barley - contains both soluble (reduces heart disease risk) and insoluble (lower risk of colon cancer) fiber, known to lower cholesterol, even better than oats, it is used in soups, breakfast cereal or as a rice substitute.

Buckwheat - is a grain that has an antioxidant that can improve circulation and is advertised to block LDL ("bad" cholesterol). It is known as "soba" noodles, and the flour makes a yummy gluten-free crepe.

Bulgar - is good source of fiber, protein, iron and vitamin B-6. Eating whole-grain foods, including bulgur, may lower the risk of developing cardiovascular disease, according to the Harvard School of Public Health.

Kamut - is high in vitamin E, which is good for the skin. It's also high in magnesium, which has been shown to lower the risk of type II diabetes. It's known as flatbread and porridge.

Quinoa - is known as the best source of plant protein, contains all essential amino acids, plus folic acid, should rinse before cooking to wash away saponins, a bitter residue the plant uses to ward off insects.

Rye - is high in fiber, good for diabetics due to its low glycemic index, great grain for people trying to lose weight.

Spelt - is easily digestible, high in B vitamins, especially riboflavin, which can help reduce frequency of migraines, higher in protein than regular wheat. People who are gluten sensitive may tolerate this grain, excellent source of manganese (essential for bone health and glucose metabolism).

Teff - has a poppy seed-like texture, sweet, molasses flavored, and high in fiber, iron, and calcium. Used as a flour in many baked goods.

Wheat Berries – is the most natural form of original whole grain, Great source of manganese, magnesium, selenium and phosphorus, contains lignans, which may help to protect against breast and prostate cancer. It's used in soups, muffins, breads and salads. [4]

BEANS

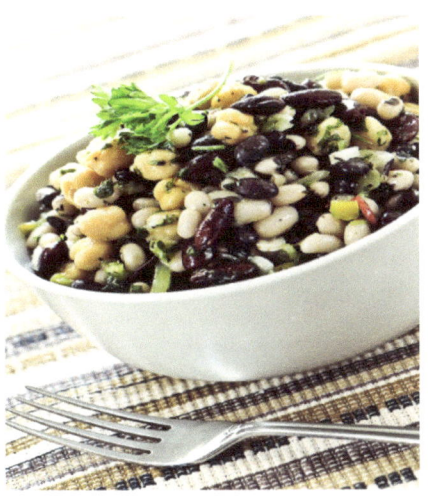

According to Dr. Fuhrman, *Beans Protect against Colon Cancer* [5], beans help protect against colon cancer and stabilize blood sugar. There are chickpeas, black-eyed peas, kidney, pinto, great northern, and many other types of beans including lima beans, which just happen to be the bean with the highest content of vitamin B. B vitamins are essential for growth and the development of many bodily functions. Other important benefits include, easing anxiety and stress, supporting memory and boosting energy.

OILS

No Heat to Low Temperature Oils

Unrefined oils require no or low heat and are highly valued for their full-bodied flavor, enticing aroma, deep color, and richer nutrient content. Examples are flaxseed oil, extra virgin olive oil, and unrefined walnut and hazelnut oils.

Olive Oil has a low smoke point so it should only be used to cook at low temperatures. It can add a great flavor to slow-roast vegetables in the oven. Olive oil is a tasty oil, perfect (and common) as a salad dressing.

Extra-Virgin Olive Oil is a monounsaturated fat and research shows that monounsaturated fats help keep "bad" LDL cholesterol low and boost levels of "good" HDL cholesterol. In addition, extra-virgin olive oil is high in antioxidants called polyphenols that have been linked to heart health. "Pure" olive oil (not virgin) doesn't contain these "bonus" antioxidant.

Flaxseed Oil is highly unstable, and must be stored in the refrigerator in dark glass. When heated, it quickly becomes rancid which can cause oxidative damage to your cells. Flaxseed oil is high in omega-3 essential fat, and should be poured over salads.

Medium to High Temperature Oils

Refined oils are actually the better choice for cooking at medium to high temperatures. Refined oils include canola oil, refined peanut oil, high oleic safflower oil, refined sesame oil, and refined coconut oil.

High Temperature Oils

Coconut Oil refined is the most stable oil for cooking. It is anti-bacterial, antiviral and is an antioxidant. It's also high in lauric acid, which is the saturated fat found in breast milk.

Avocado Oil also has a high smoke point. It has a light nutty flavor and can be used in stir-fries and when pan frying or searing fish and meat.

OILS TO AVOID

Foods that are cooked with hydrogenated oils are processed to prolong shelf life, and refined using bleaching clays and deodorizers. These processes remove all minor ingredients as well as extend the shelf life, and make the oil toxic and hard to digest.[6] Examples of the foods that are prepared using hydrogenated oils are frostings, ice cream, donuts, margarines, non-dairy coffee creamers and white bread. Remember to always check your labels for ingredients.

Plant-Based Saturated Fats Vs Animal-Based Saturated Fats

Coconut oil does contain a large amount of saturated fat, but the plant-based saturated fat found in unrefined coconut oil is different from the saturated fat found in animal foods. It's very important to understand not all fats are created equal, just as all saturated fats are not created equal. Just as there are "good fats" and "bad fats", there are also "good saturated fats" and "bad saturated fats".

Unrefined whole coconut meat, coconut milk and extra virgin coconut oil are "good saturated fats" and have a different biochemical makeup than the saturated fats found in animal foods.

Epidemiological studies show that saturated fats found in animal foods (butter, beef, dairy, turkey, chicken, eggs) can be harmful to heart health. However, the saturated fat found in unrefined and unprocessed coconut foods is not harmful.

For years, many people have been grouping all saturated fats together and have been blaming all saturated fats for increasing the risk of heart disease. Population studies of people living in the Pacific Islands and Asia, whose diets are naturally very high in unrefined coconut foods, show surprisingly low incidences of cardiovascular disease. [7]

PROTEINS

Growing up, I thought that proteins only came from animal products. This was a problem for me since I was not a huge meat eater. There were however, some meats that I loved and could not do without.

As I've gotten older, I found that my body really does not crave or desire meat as it did when I was younger. As I continued to mature as a young woman, I learned that I could get proteins from various sources. Some healthy protein choices which I have discovered include quinoa, beans, nuts, chia seeds and other fruits and vegetables.

Personally, I was never a big bean eater either, which is a popular source of protein. Don't get me wrong, I love beans, but they have not always agreed with my digestive system. I actually ate them in limited quantities. My discovery was that I wasn't cooking them properly. It is best to soak them before cooking them; the length of time depends on the beans. The health benefits of proteins include nutrients that are needed by your body such as minerals and fiber.

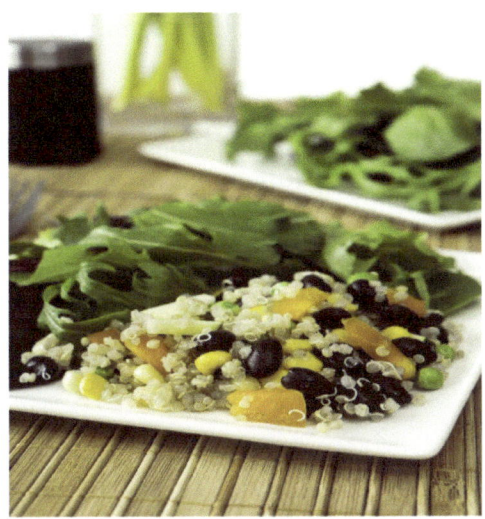

Protein in Legumes: Garbanzo beans, kidney beans, lentils, lima beans, navy beans, soybeans, split peas

Protein in Grains: Barley, brown rice protein, buckwheat, millet, oatmeal, quinoa, rye, wheat germ, wheat, wild rice

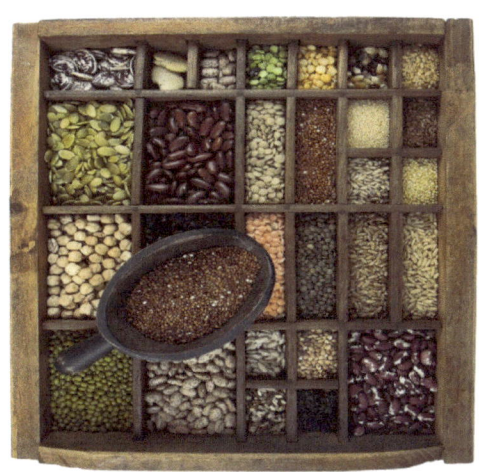

Protein in Vegetables: Artichokes, beets, broccoli, brussel sprouts, cabbage, cauliflower, cucumbers, eggplant, green peas, green pepper, kale, lettuce, mushroom, mustard

green, onions, potatoes, spinach, tomatoes, turnip greens, watercress, yams, zucchini

Protein in Fruits: Apple, banana, cantaloupe, grape, grapefruit, honeydew melon, orange, papaya, peach, pear, pineapple, strawberry, tangerine, watermelon

Protein in Nuts and Seeds: Almonds, cashews, filberts, hemp seeds, peanuts, pumpkin seeds, sesame seeds, sunflower seeds, walnuts (black)

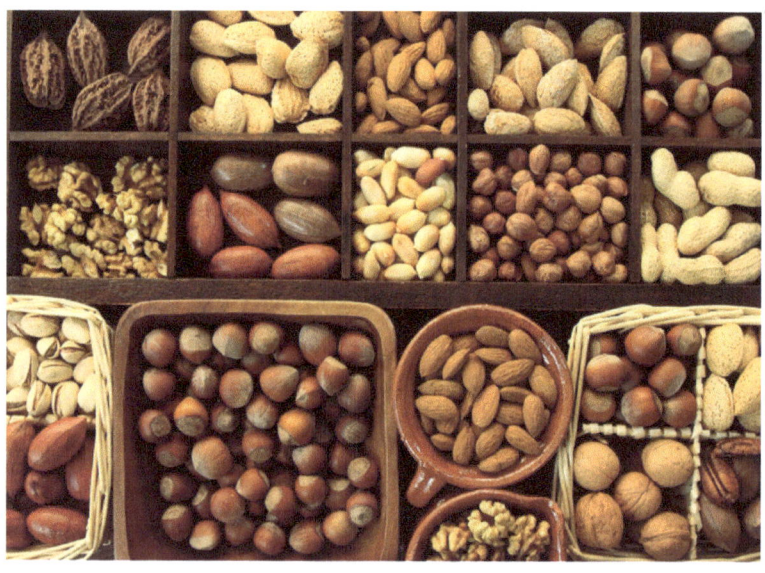

PROTECT YOUR BONES

The Trio of Calcium, Vitamin D and K can protect your bones.

Calcium is important for strong bones, teeth and much more. The more common forms of calcium are cheese, yogurt, milk, and sardines.

A sample list of Dairy Free Forms of Calcium are dark leafy greens, seafood, legumes, fruit, tofu, chia seeds, bok choy, figs, white beans, spinach, sesame seeds, and almonds. If you eat non-dairy sources of calcium it is important to pair them with vitamin D and K.

Vitamin D increases absorption of calcium, so the body receives the full benefit, while vitamin K helps make sure calcium builds up in the bones and not in tissues. That is why Vitamins D and K are essential vitamins for the proper absorption of calcium.

A sample list of Vitamin D Foods is maitake, portabella, chanterelle, and oyster mushrooms, plus, fortified soymilk, orange juice, yogurt, eggs and cheese. Vitamin D is referred to as the sunshine vitamin. When we are outside, the sun uses our body to make vitamin D.

Vitamin K is found in green leafy vegetables such as cabbage, turnip greens, broccoli, lettuce, and spinach. Green tea is another good source of Vitamin K, and one cup gives you your daily requirement of this nutrient.

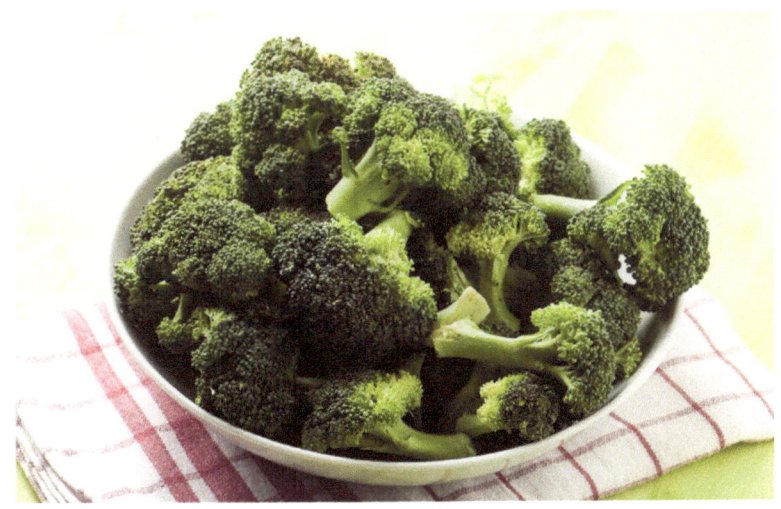

Every positive thought
is a silent prayer which will change your life.

~Bryant McGill

CHAPTER 3
HAVE MORE ENERGY

As a young child, I remember having so much energy that I could go from early morning to late night without taking a break or stopping. As I've gotten older, it seems like my energy level has decreased; I thought that it was age related. I thought that as I got older, I was supposed to have less energy and not be as active as I was in my younger days. However, I've learned that the body does change but we can change along with the body.

Being aware of which foods give the body energy is one of the keys to maintaining proper energy levels. I have learned to eat certain foods that give my body energy. If I choose mainly healthy foods, I feel more alive. If I choose processed foods and foods cooked with improper oils; it's hard to digest. When I combine processed foods, foods cooked with improper oils and sugary foods I have noticed a decrease in my energy level; which lets me know that as I have gotten older, I do not have to have less energy. The key to maintaining a stable energy level is proper nutrition.

It all boils down to the choices we make and the food we put into our bodies.

Suggestions to have more energy daily

1. Eat meals with a low glycemic load. The glycemic load is the impact in which carbohydrate containing foods affect our blood sugar. Combine whole grains and vegetables (high fiber foods) with a moderate amount of good fats and lean protein.

2. Eat foods rich in B vitamins, such as whole grains, and nutritional yeast, an inactive yeast that is favored among vegans.

3. Eat just the right amount and type of protein for your body – keep a food journal to observe how protein works best for you.

4. Stay hydrated – dehydration often causes fatigue and headache.

5. Avoid caffeine, which worsen blood sugar fluctuation.

6. Eat a calcium-rich food for your major meal of the day (leafy greens). Calcium has a soothing effect on the nervous system. This will reduce toxins in the body, can help minimize brain fog, and boost the immune system, which can increase energy. It can also help improve digestion, absorption and the assimilation of nutrients, making them more available to support daily activities.

CHAPTER 4
READ YOUR LABELS

I was not aware of the importance of reading labels until my research. The food industry can be misleading to the consumer.

As a parent, I feel the food industry is misleading parents by creating cartoon boxes for cereals with "whole grain" stamped on them. What they don't tell you is that the cereal also contains 10 grams of sugar per serving.

Reading the ingredients listed on a nutrition label can be intimidating at times. Here are a few things to keep in mind when you look at an ingredient list:

Ingredients are listed in order from the greatest amount to the least. The fewer the number of ingredients, the better.

The first or second ingredient should be what the packaging claims the product to be. If the first ingredient is "sugar", put it back! If the first ingredient says "enriched wheat flour"… think twice. If there's a long list of ingredients you can't pronounce, it is not a good idea to purchase the product.

Say no to artificial sweeteners, colorings and flavorings – they are not good for our overall health.

What's On the Box? Beware of Front Label

What some food manufacturers put on their packaging can be confusing at times. They can give consumers a false sense of eating healthy; leading them to eat more processed and packaged foods, which can lead to health problems that we have seen increase each year. For example, the term "whole grain" is allowed to be used very loosely. The basic nutritional value of flour made from whole grain is quite different from eating the whole grain in its entirety – such as cooked quinoa, brown rice, or millet.

Other areas to consider when reading food labels are:

1. *Fortified, enriched, added, extra, and plus* = nutrients such as minerals and fiber have been removed and vitamins added in processing.
   Look for 100% whole-wheat bread, and high-fiber, low-sugar cereals.

2. *Fruit drink* = probably little or no real fruit and lots of sugar.
   Look for products that say "100% Fruit Juice", and consume in moderation. Even better, eat a piece of fruit instead.

3. *Made with wheat, rye, or multi-grains* = have very little whole grain.
   Look for the word "whole" before the grain to ensure that you're getting a 100% whole-grain product.

4. *Natural* = the manufacturer started with a natural source, but once it's processed the food may not resemble anything natural.
   Look for "100% All Natural" and "No Preservatives."[8]

Food labels tell you what's in the package. Reading your food labels will help you make better food choices.

CHAPTER 5
NO MORE SUGAR BLUES

From childhood to adulthood, I *loved* sugary foods. I was a candy lover. As I got older, I continued to seek out foods that had sugar as a major ingredient. I used sugar based treats as rewards for myself. I would get a candy bar or a doughnut or a muffin to reward myself when something great happened.

I would even get the same sugary foods when something not so good happened to lift my spirits. Sugary foods were used to give me more energy. Growing up, I also had occasional migraine headaches and a short attention span. I have learned a lot about sugar during my wellness journey. Research has led me to facts connecting excessive energy and attention span irregularities to sugar.

Now that I have changed my eating habits and reduced the amount and the kinds of sugar that I eat, I have noticed a significant improvement in my health. Sugar comes in so many forms, therefore, reading the label of a product is very important to make sure that you are not eating sugar disguised under a different name.

Some sugar facts:

Did you know that one 12 oz can of Coke equals 39 g of sugar, which equals approximately 10 teaspoons of sugar? It is important to remember that one-teaspoon of sugar equals four grams. Sugar is a major contributor to many health conditions such as diabetes, arthritis, skin disorders, and headaches, just to name a few.

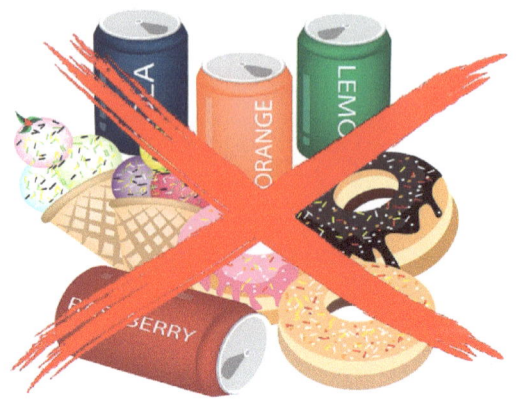

EAT LESS SUGAR, FEEL ALIVE

Avoiding refined sugar is one of the best ways to minimize blood sugar spikes and crashes, which causes a drastic change in energy level, not to mention mood swings.

The most effective way to get off sugar is to get to the root cause of your sugar cravings. Here are a few strategies:

1. Eat sweet vegetables, such as carrots, parsnips, corn, winter squash, sweet potatoes and onion to satisfy your body's need for sweet tasting foods.

2. Eat meals with a low glycemic load. When the crash approaches; don't reach for sugar for a quick fix. Combine whole grains and vegetables (high fiber foods) with a moderate amount of good fats and lean protein.

3. Stay hydrated – thirst is sometimes mistaken as hunger, which leads to cravings.

4. Make sure you are eating foods that are providing the most nutrients to your body and not junk foods. (*See your health care professional*)

5. Nourish your soul – some people crave sweets out of boredom or loneliness.

WHAT'S WRONG WITH SUGAR

Sugar addiction can result in many health issues for you that affect your overall health and wellbeing. It is important to be informed and make the best health decisions.

Refined table sugar, which is processed, is called sucrose; it is extracted from either sugar cane or beets and then refined. During the process, it is stripped of its vitamins, minerals, and fiber. It actually requires extra effort from the body to digest and assimilate. The body must deplete its own store of minerals and enzymes to absorb sucrose properly.

Therefore, instead of providing the body with nutrients, refined sugar creates deficiencies. Sugar has lots of negative health consequences. It can suppress the immune system, weaken eyesight, cause hypoglycemia, cause weight gain, exacerbate arthritis, contribute to the development of osteoporosis, increase cholesterol, lead to prostate and ovarian cancer, contribute to the development of diabetes, speed up skin aging, increase fluid retention, cause poor concentration, and lead to mood swings and depression. [7]

If sugar causes us so much trouble, why are we still hooked?

The primary reason is that sugar is an addictive substance because:

1. Eating even a small amount creates a desire for more; and,
2. Sudden quitting causes withdrawal symptoms such as headaches, mood swings, cravings and fatigue. [9]

THE MANY NAMES OF SUGAR

So you know eating sugar is bad for you, but do you know how to identify all forms of sugar that will cause just as much concern as plain "sugar"? Here are the different names that sugar may appear as in foods.
- Brown sugar, confectioners sugar, powdered sugar
- Cane juice/evaporated cane juice
- Corn syrups
- Dextrose, or glucose, aka corn sugar
- High-fructose corn syrup (HFCS)
- Honey
- Lactose or milk sugar
- Laevulose or fructose
- Raw sugar
- Sorbitol, mannitol, malitol and xylitol (sugar alcohol)
- Sucrose or table sugar [10]

ARTIFICIAL SWEETENERS

What about using artificial sweeteners to satisfy your sweet tooth? They contain zero calories.

Artificial sweeteners may taste like sugar, but your body doesn't recognize them as food. They are chemicals that your body recognize as toxins, and add to your body's toxic load. Symptoms of toxicity can include: fatigue, headache, mood changes, digestive issues and brain fog.

Studies have found that the sweet taste without the calories actually alters our perception of satiety – we are telling our brain that sweet taste no longer equates to calories. Research has shown that people who consume diet drinks and use artificial sweeteners actually gain weight, instead of lose weight.

Here are some common artificial sweeteners that you should look out for when reading food labels. It pays to become familiar with both their generic/chemical name, as well as the brand names that are used in marketing to make sure you don't miss any of them:

- Aspartame, sold under the brand names NutraSweet® and Equal® contain a neurotoxin
- Saccharin, sold under the brand name Sweet'N Low®
- Sucralose, sold under the brand name Splenda®
- Acesulfame K (or acesulfame potassium), produced by Hoechst, a German chemical company; widely used in foods, beverages and pharmaceutical products around the world.
- Neotame, produced by the NutraSweet Company, is the most recent addition to FDA's list of approved artificial sweeteners; neotame is used in diet soft drinks and low-calorie foods.[11]

Other sugars options are: maple syrup grade B and date sugar.

WAYS TO KEEP YOUR BLOOD SUGAR STEADY

1. Eat a quality breakfast
Eat a high quality protein breakfast. Good choices include: eggs, a protein shake, or oatmeal. If you opt for oatmeal or another grain, make sure to add some nuts and good quality fat such as coconut oil or almond butter for more sustainable energy.

2. Plan your meals ahead of time
Lunch should include a good quality protein and vegetables, and perhaps a small portion of a healthy grain such as quinoa or brown rice.

3. Graze
Keep healthy snacks stashed in a desk drawer, in a small cooler pack, in your bag or backpack, or even the glove

compartment of your car. Grazing on healthy foods will keep your blood sugar steady, and will actually help you control your weight much more effectively than skipping meals or snacks only to binge when your blood sugar crashes.

4. Keep an emergency food stash on hand
• A small bag of raw almonds, walnuts, cashews, and other nuts or a nuts and seed combination are also great choices. A serving size is a small handful.
• For variety and flavor you can mix the nuts and seeds with some crumbled toasted nori or dulse both are super nutritious and tasty seaweeds.
• An apple or orange.
• A small container of almond butter to eat on a sliced apple.
• A small bar of 70% dark chocolate (cacao); a serving is 1-2 squares.

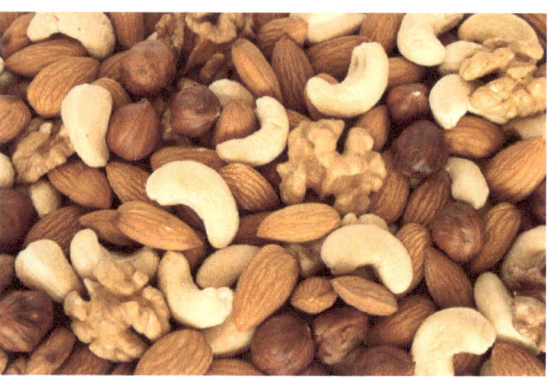

Other excellent snack choices include a small container of sliced vegetables and hummus, a hard-boiled egg, and healthy trail mix (raw almonds, walnuts, goji berries, shredded dried unsweetened coconut, dark chocolate chips).
12

CHAPTER 6
NUTRITIOUS SNACKS

Growing up, my favorite snacks were candies, chips, sodas, and french fries. They were those good sweet and salty snacks that came in plastic bags and I could buy at the corner store. There was no thought given to eating a healthy snack, it was just a "snack". Anything that tasted sweet or salty or crunchy were my favorites.

As I've gotten older and wiser, I realize that the snacks that I was eating were causing illness in my body and weight gain. Truth be told, I felt that I couldn't stop eating them even if I wanted to stop. It was like my body craved the sweet, salty, and crunchy snacks.

The more foods that I ate, found in a bag or wrapper, from the corner store; the more my body started to crave them, and I couldn't stop eating. It was like they were calling my name whenever I passed them in the store. The results, however, were extra body weight, feeling sluggish, tired, skin breakouts, and warnings from my doctor that I needed to improve my diet.

LIST OF HEALTHY SNACKS

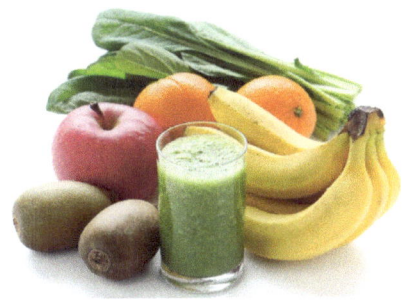

Cut vegetables, fruits, smoothies, nuts, hemp hearts, kale chips, chia seeds, avocado and bananas in a pudding are among my favorite snacks.

BAD MOOD FOODS

Alcohol, candy bars, fast food, junk food, chips, soda and coffee top the list of bad mood foods. If a food is high in sugar, salt, caffeine, excess fat or artificial ingredients, it could have a negative effect on how you feel. Sugar, for example, affects your mood hormones and insulin levels. Alcohol is a depressant. And though these things may make you feel better temporarily, you'll end up feeling worse in the long run.

CHAPTER 7
SUPER FOODS FOR A SUPER BODY

Superfoods are foods that fill a nutritional deficiency. When you eat sugar, refined carbs, or transfats your body gets robbed of nutrients. The body has to pull on its reserves in order to break down these foods. Superfoods do just the opposite. They provide an abundance of nutrients and act to fill in the gaps so you feel more energized, your skin glows, you think better, digestion improves, and you simply feel more alive.

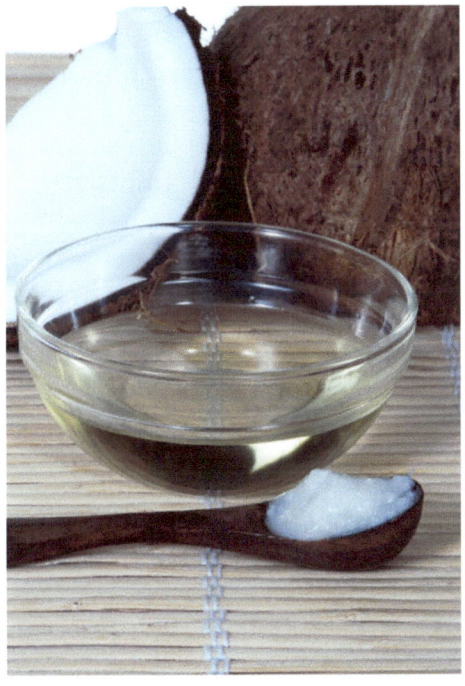

Coconut Oil
- High In Electrolytes: potassium, magnesium, phosphorous, sodium, and calcium
- Directly lowers blood pressure in 71% of people

- Hydrates your skin from the inside, heals acne scars burns fat, has anti-viral, anti-fungal, and antibacterial properties

Raw Cacao
- Contains Arginine, which plays an important role in the release of hormones in the body
- Contains the compound phenylethylamine and anandamide, which makes us feel "blissed out"
- High in chromium which balances blood sugar
- High in B vitamins, which helps you stay sharp and focused
- High in magnesium which supports heart health, relieves menstrual cramps, and increases alkalinity

Dark Leafy Greens
- Loaded with iron, calcium, potassium, and magnesum plus vitamins, including vitamins K, C, E and many of the B vitamins
- High in phytonutrients, which keeps your eyes healthy
- High dose of Vitamin K protects your bones from osteoporosis

Raw Goji Berries
- Elevates mood, 14% protein, and the highest food in the world in beta carotene (more than carrots!)
- Vitamin C is 50 times greater than the amount in oranges, contains 21 trace minerals, and polysaccharides, which fortify the immune system
- Stimulates the body to naturally produce growth hormone

Hemp Seed
- High in protein
- Contains all 20 amino acids that sustain life

- High in fiber, which keeps things moving in your GI tract
- Boosts immune system
- Easily digestible

Flaxseed
- High in omega 3's - "good" fats that have been shown to have heart-healthy effects
- Lignans have both plant estrogen and antioxidant qualities. Each tablespoon of ground flaxseed contains about 1.8 grams of plant omega-3s
- High in fiber

Chia Seeds
- Rich in antioxidants, vitamin c, omega 3 and 6
- High in fiber
- High in protein
- High in calcium, phosphorous, magnesium, manganese, copper, iron, molybdenum, niacin, and zinc

Super Foods slow the absorption of sugar giving you more long-lasting energy without the crash [13]

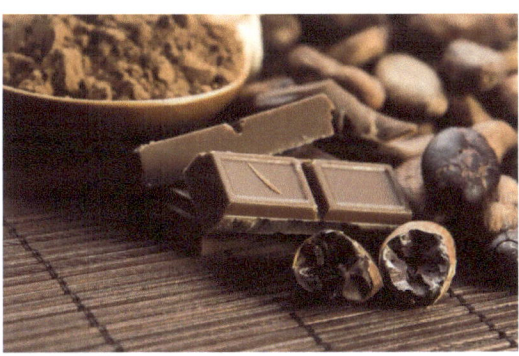

Let food be thy medicine, and
let medicine be thy food.

~Hippocrates

CHAPTER 8
WHAT'S THE DIFFERENCE: DETOX, CLEANSING AND FASTING

You hear so much these days about detoxing, cleansing and fasting. People often ask, "Are they the same and should I do all three. When should I use them and how often?"

Detox has been a hot topic and it's not just for the super-health-conscious folks or people who eat only quinoa and kale anymore. Toxins affect all of us and just by changing a few things to clean up your life, you can see a dramatic difference in your health and wellbeing. The question is no longer IF we are toxic, but HOW toxic are you?

Detoxification is a process during which you normalize the body's natural ability to process and excrete toxins that are stored in our fat, while temporarily reducing the amount of incoming toxins. When eating foods that provide the vitamins, nutrients, and antioxidants that the body needs for detoxification, such as high fiber foods and water; toxins are eliminated by increasing the frequency of bowel movements and urination. A detox may be preferred if there has been some over exposure to chemicals, medication or alcohol.[14]

Cleansing is basically the same as a detox, however, a cleanse is more of a general form of detoxification where you focus on the liver, colon or kidneys. [15] A cleansing program is used when the body gives you signs that it is either sick or feeling slow and sluggish, or as a preventative maintenance. Specific foods to eat on a cleansing program will depend on your focus. Generally you will eat high fiber foods such as fruits, vegetables, nuts, seeds, legumes and herbs. Foods to avoid during a cleanse are sugar, chocolate, alcohol, caffeinated products, animal protein, milk, dairy, poultry and seafood.

Fasting is refraining from certain foods or drinks for a certain period of time. According to Dr. Hass [16] one should take a break from the big five: sugar, alcohol, wheat, dairy and caffeine for a period of 1-3 weeks. You decide what is best for you but it is good to give your body a break from food for even a short period. Always consult your doctor.

So, how toxic we are? Sometimes symptoms of toxicity can be quite non-specific and therefore hard to pin down. We are all different genetically, so we react to toxins differently and at different dosages. Toxic exposure can manifest itself very differently in different people. If you have health issues that have been lingering for a while, it's worth looking at toxicity being the root cause.

Common symptoms of excessive toxic burden can include:
- Fatigue
- Depression
- Headaches
- Cognitive problems: brain fog, memory problems
- Neurological issues: balance problems, tremors [17]

5 SIMPLE WAYS TO REDUCE YOUR TOXIC EXPOSURE

I have cured myself of some joint aches and headache symptoms by eliminating chemicals from my life. I have seen improvement not only in my energy level, but also from my family members by cleaning up our diet and environment.

Reducing your toxic exposure can lead to many health benefits, including: weight loss, clear skin, mental acuity, reduced stress, more energy, improved immune function, better digestion and reduced food cravings.

Here are 5 tips to reduce your toxic load:

1. An aerobic exercise that causes you to sweat.

2. Using herbs that support detoxing the organs such as milk thistle, and dandelion.

3. Reduce processed and packaged foods, which are loaded with chemicals.

4. Replace household and personal products loaded with chemicals with those made with natural ingredients.

5. Buy and eat organic food as much as possible – learn about the "Dirty Dozen" list and try to shop organic for these produce. [18]

12 Most Contaminated / Dirty Dozen™

1. Apples
2. Celery
3. Strawberries
4. Peaches
5. Spinach
6. Nectarines (Imported)
7. Grapes (Imported)
8. Sweet bell peppers
9. Potatoes
10. Blueberries (Domestic)
11. Lettuce
12. Kale / Collard greens

15 Least Contaminated / Clean 15™

1. Onions
2. Corn
3. Pineapples

4. Avocado
5. Asparagus
6. Sweet Peas
7. Mangoes
8. Eggplant
9. Cantaloupe
10. Kiwi
11. Cabbage
12. Watermelon
13. Sweet potatoes
14. Grapefruit
15. Mushrooms

There are many detox programs available with varying lengths and ingredients. Find the one that appeals to you and your lifestyle. You and your health care provider can determine which is best for you. If you have a high toxic load, you will release a high level of toxins from your body. Using a detox procedure without prior experience or proper supervision can create a counter reaction. Remember the following:

• Severe detox symptoms including headache, lethargy, and skin reactions
• When looking for a safe detox protocol and program pay special attention to a gradual approach that can minimize withdrawal, sudden toxin release, and increase your success rate
• Take in enough calories to support the body's detoxification and elimination process
• Address issues of addiction prior to starting any program

When you are looking to start a weight loss program, it's best to go through a supervised detox program first so fewer problems will arise when toxins are released as fat cells are burned off.

CHAPTER 9
PROCESS OF ELIMINATION: DIGESTIVE HEALTH

Natural Ways to Facilitate Elimination

Having previously suffered from slow digestive issues for some time, I healed myself using nutrition and lifestyle changes. Digestive issues can be very inconvenient and painful, if one does not address the problem.

Constipation can be very uncomfortable and even painful, and studies have even found that infrequent bowel movements allow toxins to linger in the colon, increasing the risk of developing cancer.

Here are a few ways to get things moving:

1. Drink a cup of warm water with the juice of half a lemon when you get up in the morning. It is very cleansing, aids liver function and moves the bile.

2. Exercise regularly – body movements help digestion.

3. Drink the fresh juice of carrots and apples to aid colon detox. Raw is best because the enzymes present also aid digestion.

4. Ensure adequate intake of dietary fiber – fruits, vegetables, whole grains, flaxseed, wheat bran and chia seeds.

Relieve Gas Safely and Effectively

Having gas can be uncomfortable and embarrassing. There is something that you can do to ease the discomfort and bloating that is associated with gas. The most common reasons are food intolerance and too much fiber all at once.

Talking and chewing at the same time also allows excessive air to enter the stomach. This is an important reason to pay attention to your eating habits.

Here are a few ways to safely get rid of bloating through nutritional and holistic approaches:
• Use herbs such as basil, dill, ginger, fennel, and mint as tea or in your cooking- all of these herbs have gas-relieving properties.
• Introduce fiber-rich food gradually - fiber is great, but too much in the diet and suddenly eating a lot of fiber-rich food will cause your GI tract to resist it.
• Cook beans properly - soak beans, and use spices to improve digestibility.
• Notice how your body reacts to vegetables such as broccoli and cabbage, and use moderate intake if necessary.
• Look for potential food intolerance (e.g. lactose or gluten) - if your body cannot digest and assimilate these nutrients properly, they can cause gas.
• Yoga poses such as twisting can help relieve gas - these poses stimulate the movement of the smooth muscles of the intestinal walls and help "move things along".

Indigestion and Poor Digestion

Indigestion is another issue that I have had to address. After writing down and being mindful of what and when I ate; I was able to heal myself with lifestyle changes. Digestive issues can be very inconvenient and painful. Indigestion and a poor digestive system can be caused by low digestive enzymes, lack of intestinal flora, poor eating habits, poor-quality foods, and stress.

Lifestyle and dietary changes help ease indigestion and improve the overall digestive process:

- Slow down when you eat
- Chew slowly and thoroughly

- Refrain from drinking immediately before or after a meal, and don't drink during the meal – this can dilute stomach acid.
- Be mindful about food combination – carbohydrates and protein can result in gas. Certain fruits ferment quickly which can occur in your stomach and should be eaten alone (melons)
- Drink ginger, peppermint or chamomile tea 30 min before and after meals
- Add ginger and cayenne to your food – use fresh-grated ginger and only a few grains of cayenne
- Use papaya enzyme to aid digestion, and supplement with acidophilus to restore healthy gut flora. [19]

Immune Support

A short list of foods that will support and increase the function of your immune system:

- Spices -- garlic, thyme, rosemary, basil, sage, oregano and others spices and herbs
- Ginger
- Onions
- Yogurt
- Mushrooms
- Garlic
- Citrus fruits are loaded with vitamin C that the body needs

Almost any food that is not processed is good for the immune system. It's the processed foods that make the body sluggish.

Keep In Mind

With thousands of diets on the market, it is hard to distinguish which one is the right diet for each individual. Diets range from primarily protein to mostly vegetables to soups and fruits. The best practice is to follow a nutrient rich diet, so that your body receives the nutrients that it needs to maintain optimal health. This will vary from person to person. Your doctor can advise you on specific health questions.

Getting and staying healthy involves the whole body. My approach to health and wellness involves the Mind, Body and Spirit. By incorporating small steps you can *Create The Life You Want and Feel Fabulous Inside and Out.* Start today!

*Knowing
is not enough;
we must apply.
Being willing
is not enough;
we must do*

~Leonardo da Vinci

Track Your Progress

Creating The Life You Want for your health takes a single thought, idea, dream or strong desire to try something new. Once you have that idea and motivation, it is time to put it into planning mode. This chart gives you a place to record your goals, steps to achieve them, and progress.

Goals	Steps	Progress
	1. 2. 3.	
	1. 2. 3.	
	1. 2. 3.	
	1. 2. 3.	

NOTES

Shopping List Guide

Creating The Life You Want for your health includes planning your meals and trying new foods. Use this shopping checklist as a guide to help you keep track of the healthy foods you purchase. Variety is important in food choices to keep your meals interesting. It is suggested that you try at least one new food in each category when shopping.

Vegetables	Grains	Beans
Fruits	Condiments	Spices
Snacks	Beverages	Other

REFERENCES

1.	Rosenthal, Joshua. *Integrative Nutrition*, Austin. Greenleaf. 2011

2.	Fuhrman, Joel. Eat To Live, New Your. Little Brown and Company. 2011.

3.	Table of vegetables from http://pforlife.com/fruits-vegetables-their-benefits.html

4.	http://www.mindbodygreen.com/0-9801/a-simple-health-guide-to-the-most-common-grains.html

5.	https://www.drfuhrman.com/library/beans_cancer.aspx

6.	http://www.mindbodygreen.com/0-7605/what-you-need-to-know-about-eating-oils.html

7.	http://www.cleancuisineandmore.com/is-the-saturated-fat-in-coconut-harmful/

8.	http://www.webmd.com/food-ecipes/features/how-read-nutrition-label

9.	http://www.all-creatures.org/health/howsugarcan.html

10.	http://www.inspirationgreen.com/all-the-different-sugars.html

11.	http://www.fitsugar.com/Side--Side-Comparisons-Artificial-Sweeteners-1133886

12.	http://www.mindbodygreen.com/0-7365/4-ways-to-keep-your-blood-sugar-steady.html

13.   http://www.mindbody.com/0-7264/8-best-superfoods-to-boost-your-mood-energy-levels.html

14.   http://www.healthy.net/scr/article.aspx?Id=1558

15.   http://www.alive.com/articles/view/23820/cleansing_and_detox_faqs

16.   http://www.elsonhaas.com/templates/haashealthcenter/images/tips/springcleaning.html

17.   http://www.livestrong.com/article/67812-signs-toxins-body/

18.   http://www.ewg.org/foodnews/summary/

19.   Gladstar, R. *Herbal Recipes for Vibrant Health*. Storey Publishing, 2008.

http://www.huffingtonpost.com/kristin-kirkpatrick-ms-rd-ld/dangers-of-sugar_b_3658061.html

https://www.moodcure.com/good_mood_foods.html

Campbell, T. C. and Esselstyn, C. B. Forks over Knives: The plant-based way to health. New York. The Experiment, LLC, 2011

Photo Credits

All photos used in this book were purchased from CanStockPhoto.com and are licensed for commercial use.

Documentaries

These documentaries are eye opening. There are many available, here are several to get you started:

Forks Over Knives
Food Matters
Hungry For Change
Food Inc.
Fat, Sick & Nearly Dead

Books

Eat to Live by Joel Fuhrman, M.D. Little, Brown and Company, 2011.

Integrative Nutrition: Feed your Hunger for Happiness by Joshua Rosenthal. Integrative Nutrition Publishing, 2011.

Thrive: The Vegan Nutrition Guide to Optimal Performance in Sports and Life by Brendan Brazier. Da Capo Press, 2007.

Forks Over Knives by T. Colin Campbell, PhD and Caldwell B. Esselstyn, Jr, M.D. The Experiment Publishing, 2011.

The Mood Cure: The 4-Step Program to Take Charge of Your Emotions-Today by Julia Ross. Penguin Books, 2002.

The Diet Cure: The 8-Step Program to Rebalance Your Body Chemistry and End Food Cravings, Weight Gain, and Mood Swings-Naturally by Julia Ross. Penguin Books, 2000.

The Blood Sugar Solution: The UltraHealthy Program for Losing Weight, Preventing Disease, and Feeling Great Now! By Mark Hyman, M.D. Hyman Enterprises, 2012.

ABOUT ANGELA BOYD

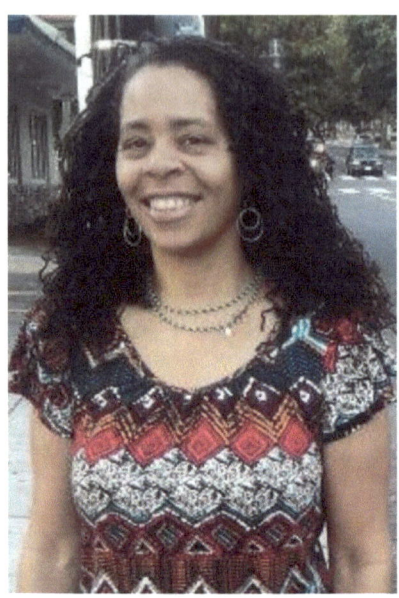

As a Certified Holistic Health Coach, and owner of Natural Health Essence Angela enjoys inspiring and encouraging others to make positive changes in their life.

Her private practice consists of coaching clients to reach their goals for health, weight loss, and stress reduction. She believes no one diet works for everyone because each person has unique food and lifestyle needs. During her training with the Institute for Integrative Nutrition (IIN), Angela studied more that 100 dietary theories and a variety of practical lifestyle coaching methods. As she draws on this knowledge, she helps clients create a completely personalized "roadmap to health" that suits each unique body, lifestyle, preferences, and set of goals. Angela presents workshops and lectures on living a healthy balanced life.

Helping her clients discover simple, natural solutions for their health is very important to Angela. Additionally, she shows you how to take care of yourself, family and friends with pure and potent oils known as essential oils. You will be surprised how these natural essential oils benefit the body.

Angela is a member of Toastmasters International and has over 20 years in counseling youth and adults in issues relating to making lifestyle choices. She is currently studying to become a yoga teacher. She is known to be well informed, current, positive, inspirational, always concerned about her clients, an excellent listener, intuitive, resourceful, and available when needed the most. Angela Boyd is the proud mother of three wonderful children and enjoys spending time with her family and friends.

Website:
http://www.NaturalHealthEssence.com/

Facebook:
https://www.facebook.com/NaturalHealthEssence

Twitter:
https://twitter.com/NHEssence

TO ORDER:

Create The Life You Want: Feel Fabulous Inside And Out

Visit
www.NaturalHealthEssence.com
or
www.Amazon.com

Book Disclaimer

This book was written to spark the desire within to make positive and possibly necessary changes to your overall health and well being.

My role as a Health Coach and author is not to prescribe or treat on any of these levels: provide health care; medical or nutrition therapy services; diagnose, treat or cure any disease, condition or other physical or mental ailment of the human body. Rather, as a Coach, I am a mentor and guide who has been trained in holistic health coaching to assist clients in reaching their own health goals as they devise and implement positive, sustainable lifestyle changes. This book is not to act in the capacity of a doctor, licensed dietician-nutritionist, psychologist or other licensed or registered professional. Any advice given is not meant to take the place of advice given by these professionals. If you are under the care of a health care professional or currently taking prescription medications, you should discuss any dietary changes or potential use of dietary supplements with your doctor, and should not discontinue any prescription medications without first consulting the doctor.